I0423506

Prepper's Survival Medicine Handbook

The Ultimate Prepper's Guide to Preparing
Emergency First Aid and Survival Medicine
for you and your Family

Timothy S. Morris
www.timothymorrisbooks.com

Table of Contents

Chapter One: An Introduction to This Guide

      What You Can Expect from This Guide

      What's the Difference Between First Aid and Survival Medicine Anyway?

Chapter Two: Basic First Aid

      The Importance of First Aid Training

      The First Aid Kit

      What Goes in a First Aid Kit Anyway?

      The Basics

      Useful Add-ons

      Location, Location, Location

      First Aid 101

      Nine Simple Steps to Properly Assess Any Situation

      Common First Aid Scenarios

      Bleeding Wounds and Other Lacerations

      Nosebleeds

      Burns

      Bites

      Sudden collapse

      Car accidents

      Frostbite and Hypothermia

Severe Bleeding

Pain Relief

Head & Neck Injuries

Stabilization of the Head and Neck

Chapter Three: CPR & Rescue Breathing

Rescue Breathing

Unconscious Choking Treatment

Cardiopulmonary Resuscitation (CPR)

Chapter Four: Survival Medicine

The Benefits of Alternative Medicine

Delivery Methods

Infusions

Decoctions

Infused Oils

Vinegars

Tinctures

Glycerites

Gels

Ointments, Salves and Balms

Creams

Common Ailments and Cures

Digestive Problems

Respiratory Problems

Dermatological Problems

Kid-specific Treatments

Muscular & Joint Problems

Emotional Problems

Top 10 Herbs You Should Be Growing Right Now

Growing Herbs at Home

Conclusion

Chapter One: An Introduction to This Guide

One of the most overlooked, yet vitally important, aspects of any survival situation is medical treatment. Following a catastrophic event, emergency medical responders will be overburdened (to say the least) and unable to respond to many calls for assistance as these departments struggle to categorize emergencies based on severity and a host of other factors that likely depend on the situation.

Even in less extreme cases, think about the last time you called 911 or had to go to the ER following an injury. How long did it take to receive treatment? Were you satisfied with the results of the medical care you paid for? And if you live in a rural area, an emergency medical response could take hours in the best of circumstances. Sprinkle in some bad weather or a regional catastrophe and the reality is that you may not receive the assistance you need in time.

It's for this reason that understanding at least the basics of both emergency first aid and survival medicine are essential to any survival plan.

What You Can Expect from This Guide

This guide has been designed as an easy reference which you can refer to in times of crisis. Everything from minor burns to treatment for broken bones is covered in the chapters below. You will learn how to perform CPR and ways to manage pain when someone becomes ill or injured. For injuries too severe to be treated effectively using the methods described in this guide, you will learn techniques to minimize additional injury and avoid the symptoms of shock until such a time that professional medical assistance can be secured.

What's the Difference Between First Aid and Survival Medicine Anyway?

One of the first things we should discuss is the difference between first aid and survival medicine. The term "first aid" is thrown around so loosely that it is often used in places where another term might be more appropriate.

To better understand what first aid is, let's discuss what first aid is not.

First aid is **not** advanced medical treatment. Although having an understanding of more advanced medical practices is certainly a helpful asset, it is by no means required for many injuries.

Even if an injury is ultimately beyond the scope of your experience, training, and supplies, first aid is still useful to prevent further damage while waiting for appropriate medical treatment.

Why is first aid so important?

Let's look at some statistics. Each year over 1 million people in the United States die from some form of heart disease. About one third of these people die from sudden cardiac arrest.

First aid techniques can often save the lives of people who suddenly fall victim to heart failure.

Heart disease is the number one cause of death in the country.

Another leading cause of death is unintentional injury. Well over 100,000 Americans die from unintentional injuries each year and a staggering 25 million are disabled as a result of their injuries.

Can first aid save all of these people? Of course not – but considering how many people are not properly trained in first aid techniques it begs the question of how much lower these statistics might be if more first responders were knowledgeable in basic medical treatment.

Advanced care such as stitches and splinting fractures is considered advanced medical care. These are tactics that should be learned but it is not within the scope of first aid.

If doctors and hospitals are no longer available, you may be responsible for administering advanced treatments but a patient must be stabilized and their condition accurately assessed before any other actions are taken.

We will define first aid as emergency care or treatment that is given to an ill or injured person before trained medical staff arrives.

If trained medical staff will not be arriving at all then you may be forced to switch roles and become a caregiver. During an emergency, however, this should not be your concern. Your concern should rest solely on stabilizing the patient and assessing immediate threats to that individual's health and well-being as a result of injury or illness.

And then there's survival medicine. Although finding a definitive answer to exactly what survival medicine is (and isn't as the case may be), a good working definition which we will apply throughout this guide is that survival medicine represents a way to provide medical attention to the sick and injured using whatever materials may be available at the time. A simple example might be using a tree branch to create a splint for a broken bone.

But survival medicine should also account for long-term scenarios. Think the end of the world, apocalyptic stuff. Even if you have a first aid kit stocked with every imaginable supply, eventually those supplies will run out. Whether we are talking about medicine, bandages or any other consumable medical item, survival medicine dictates that we think about sustainable medicine whenever possible.

In addition to learning basic outdoor survival medicine strategies, we will discuss herbal alternatives that are, at least in some cases, just as effective as modern medicine. The difference is that these remedies can be grown and made in the comfort of your own home and with a proper understanding of these basic principles, you have an unlimited supply of medicine available even if society is facing imminent collapse.

Now that we've established the basic differences between first aid and survival medicine, let's look at each in more detail. The next chapter is devoted to the basics of first aid and how these concepts apply to a variety of emergency situations.

Chapter Two: Basic First Aid

Before diving into the techniques required to perform basic first aid, there are two important topics we need to discuss. Without first understanding these concepts and how they apply to an emergency situation, we have little hope of actually helping anyone — in fact, sometimes we can unintentionally do more harm than good.

The Importance of First Aid Training

There have been many documented cases where people with good intentions have actually created more harm to a victim by trying to assist in a medical emergency without proper training.

First aid guidelines are very specific for reason. When you approach an injured person, you have no idea what the extent of their injuries might be and every precaution should be taken until the source of the injury has been positively identified.

For example, moving an individual who may have some sort of spinal injury could make the injury worse and even result in permanent paralysis. Any victim who has even the slightest chance of spinal injury should not be moved without equipment designed to stabilize the spinal column.

If you do not have any experience in first aid techniques, there are tons of free or low-cost classes available.

Every adult in your family should have at least basic first aid training and learning more advanced techniques is even better.

Training is important for a couple of reasons.

First aid knowledge has been proven to save lives. The training also provides first responders with a level of confidence not found in people without first aid training. This extra confidence often helps to mitigate the onset of panic.

If you have never seen an injured person with a hysterical loved one by their side, it is an extremely stressful situation. Most people experienced in first aid training resort to their training first and let their emotions take a backseat to the immediate issue of addressing the victim's needs.

Training increases your response time during an emergency. A difference of only a few minutes can affect whether a victim survives or succumbs to their injuries.

Without oxygen, the brain dies within six minutes. Arterial bleeding can result in death within five minutes. Lacerations can quickly become infected. Shock can even lead to death relatively quickly if not managed properly.

By knowing what to do in a given situation before it occurs, you will be able to make sound judgments quickly that can have a positive impact on the health of the victim.

The First Aid Kit

Creating a first aid kit is something that should not be taken lightly. It truly is a personalized solution that represents the equipment you are trained to use and the potential situations you are likely to encounter.

Creating the perfect first aid kit begins by assessing your first aid knowledge and that of your family members.

For instance, it doesn't make sense to have equipment in your kit that no one knows how to use (there are exceptions to this). Location also plays a role in the contents of your first aid kit.

Procuring and storing anti-venom for a king cobra bite doesn't make much sense in the United States unless you happen to have one as a pet or live near a zoo.

It would be nice to have equipment for every imaginable injury but it is simply not practical due to size constraints.

I cannot stress enough the importance of assessing your individual first aid training and filling in any gaps whenever possible.

This will be beneficial to your family and other members of your community if professional medical assistance is unavailable. Local Red Cross chapters often hold training sessions from basic first aid through specialized training for wilderness survival and other less common, but equally important, situations.

Often when people think of first aid kits, they think of the neatly packaged red zipper bags that can be purchased at a variety of retailers nationwide. These kits are inexpensive but they are also ineffective.

Look at the package of one of those kits if you are doubtful. Typically, they will have a description stating their use for cuts and scrapes, minor burns, and pain or swelling.

These ailments are uncomfortable but typically not life-threatening.

A kit like this will mostly consist of various size bandages, ointment, alcohol pads, and maybe some burn cream. Unfortunately, this will not get you very far if medical attention is hours away or if it won't be coming at all.

Recently, there have been more companies selling specialized first aid kits that offer much more than the basic one described above.

This is certainly a better option and will typically include helpful items such as an assortment of medications (OTC meds such as painkillers and antihistamines), gauze dressings, irrigation syringes, a clotting compound, and CPR accessories such as face shields or mouthpieces.

Advanced kits like this are a huge step up from the basic ones sold at the local drugstore or big-box retailers.

Despite these improvements, we need more than this to become truly resilient. The only way to accomplish this is to create your own first aid kit. This ensures your kit has everything your family needs to address anticipated situations and the unexpected alike.

What Goes in a First Aid Kit Anyway?

We are about to cover a large list of items that should be in just about every first aid kit.

By no means is this list meant to be all-inclusive.

In addition to comparing it with other lists, you should take into consideration any special medical needs that may be required for you or a member of your family.

Also note that the list does not include quantities because for many items the quantity will be dictated by the number of people in your family and any other people that the kit is designed to serve.

The Basics

First Aid reference manual – You aren't expected to be knowledgeable in every situation so this manual can serve as a guide for those situations which you may not be intimately familiar with.

Gloves – At least two pairs of both latex and nitrile gloves. This avoids any complications from a latex allergy while protecting against contamination and blood-borne diseases. If you can only choose one, go with nitrile.

CPR barrier – These come in a few different forms and are designed to protect against disease transmission. Even though you may not be concerned about contracting diseases from other family members, it also makes CPR easier when blood or other bodily fluids make creating an airtight seal difficult.

Large cloth dressings – These dressings should be at least 5" x 9" (larger is better because they can always be cut to size). These are used to control bleeding from lacerations or puncture wounds.

Sterile gauze pads – Gauze should be available in a variety of sizes and has many uses including stopping bleeding and dressing wounds.

Roll bandages – Also used to dress wounds and can be cut to size as needed.

Compression bandages – Sometimes referred to as Ace bandages, these can be used to treat sprained joints. Consider having a couple of different sizes to effectively wrap various joints.

Band-Aids – These self-adhesive bandages are useful for addressing minor wounds to prevent exposure and possible infection.

Butterfly bandages – Adhesive strips that can be used to close lacerations.

Medical tape – Tape has many uses in first aid including dressing wounds, securing bandages, and holding medical equipment in place.

Triangular bandages – These are used to immobilize dislocations and fractures.

Q-tips – These are commonly used to clean wounds and to apply ointments or salves.

Sharp scissors – Shears can be used to cut bandages or victims clothing.

Wooden tongue depressors – Useful for checking for throat obstructions and can also be used to split small fractures.

Tweezers – Many uses including splinter removal. Believe it or not, splinters can turn into serious infections if left untreated.

Sewing needle – These can be used to dislodge foreign matter from underneath the skin.

Small flashlight – A small, handheld pen style flashlight can be held in the mouth to provide light while working and to examine body orifices.

Oral thermometer – Thermometers quickly diagnose fevers which could be a symptom of other, more serious conditions.

Irrigation syringe – Alternatively, you can also use a squeeze bottle. Either way it should be filled with sterile water and can be used to clean debris and excess bodily fluids out of wounds.

Splinting material – Available in a variety of materials, splinting material can usually be cut to size and secured to a limb for immobilizing dislocations and fractures.

Emergency blanket – These are useful in cold weather or when serious injury has caused the victim to go into shock. Keeping a victim warm prevents shock from becoming more serious.

Instant hot/cold packs – Having a few of each of these can help alleviate swelling and pain associated with muscle strain.

Plastic bags – Resealable plastic bags can be used to dispose of contaminated medical waste. They can also be used as makeshift irrigation devices by poking a hole in a corner.

Eye solution – A saline-based eye solution helps to irrigate debris from the eye and prevent further contamination.

Antibacterial soap – Used to clean wounds, your hands, and anything else that gets dirty or contaminated. Items that have been potentially contaminated by bodily fluids should further be sterilized using Betadine, alcohol, or heat.

Antiseptic solution – Betadine comes in liquid form and on pre-saturated pads and can be used to sterilize the area around the wound. It can also be used to purify small amounts of water for consumption.

Antibiotic ointment – This is commonly used to reduce the risk of infection to open wounds by placing it on and around the wound prior to bandaging.

Hydrocortisone cream – This cream is a topical steroid that helps the body recover from insect bites or stings and minor rashes.

Burn gel – The painkilling properties of these topical gels can help to alleviate pain caused by burned skin.

Ibuprofen – Commonly marketed as Motrin, ibuprofen is an anti-inflammatory and analgesic.

Antihistamine tablets – Products such as Benadryl can alleviate the symptoms associated with mild allergic reactions and skin irritations.

QuikClot – A blood clotting powder such as QuikClot can be used to help slow down or stop severe bleeding.

Pen and paper – These are used to record a victim's vital signs. This information can be used to keep track of progress or deterioration and also given to professional medical staff if and when they do arrive.

Hand sanitizer – This can be used to clean your hands when water is not available. Since most of them are alcohol-based, refrain from using them in open wounds whenever possible as this will be extremely uncomfortable for the victim.

Super glue – Super glue has many uses in a first aid setting. It can be used as an invisible bandage for small cuts, blisters, and abrasions. It acts as a waterproof bandage for smaller lacerations. Super glue can also be used to close larger lacerations in lieu of stitches.

This list represents the bare minimum that every kit should include. The next section represents items that are not necessary for basic first aid but could become invaluable in a more serious situation.

Useful Add-ons
Burn kit – Our basic list above include some basic equipment for addressing burns but for a more complete solution, consider adding a purpose built burn kit.

These are more appropriate for treating very serious burns or when burns are located on multiple areas of the body.

Snakebite kit – Typically, these kits include an extractor pump designed to pull venom from pooled areas in the body. It is not effective at extracting venom that has already entered the circulatory system.

Israeli Battle Dressing – These dressings are specially designed to be ultraportable and provide excellent treatment for serious hemorrhaging wounds.

Stethoscope – These can be used to verify breathing and heartbeat as well as to diagnose some respiratory issues.

Cervical collar – These are designed to immobilize the neck. One of these should be placed on a victim any time there is a possibility of neck, back, or spine injury to avoid further damage and possible paralysis.

Foldable stretcher – The folding varieties are relatively small and can be used to carry victims unable to walk on their own. Alternatively, a makeshift stretcher can usually be made from materials that are lying around.

Blood pressure cuff – These are useful for quickly determining a victim's blood pressure. Drops in blood pressure without visible hemorrhaging may point to internal bleeding or another problem.

Sutures – These are used to close serious wounds.

Locking forceps – These can be used during suturing and also can stop hemorrhaging blood vessels.

Automated External Defibrillator (AED) – These battery-operated units are very simple to use and can restart a failed heart during cardiac arrest.

Scalpel – A surgical grade scalpel can be used for minor surgery or to remove excess tissue.

Now our first aid kit is starting to show promise.

If you take the time to assemble everything just listed (and learn how to use it if necessary), you possess a formidable tool for medical treatment at home.

Next, we will look at some common medications that should be included as well. Keep in mind that some of these medications are OTC like the ibuprofen already mentioned while others require a doctor's prescription.

For prescription medications, many doctors are willing to prescribe extra medication for your first aid kit if you explain your intentions first. This will not include controlled substances such as opioid-based painkillers or other regulated medications.

Asthma inhalers – If you or someone in your family suffers from asthma, you probably already have quite a few of these lying around. Be sure to put at least one or two into your first aid kit and leave them there.

Nitroglycerin – This is commonly prescribed as a treatment for patients with heart conditions.

Aspirin – In addition to being an effective OTC painkiller, aspirin is also used to treat certain heart conditions.

Sugar pills – These can be administered to quickly bring up the blood sugar of a diabetic patient.

Insulin – If a diabetic lives in your house, make sure your kit includes a good supply of insulin and needles to administer it.

Imodium – Imodium or similar is often used to treat diarrhea. Although diarrhea may seem like more of an inconvenience, it can actually lead to severe dehydration if left unchecked.

EpiPen – These are commonly prescribed to individuals prone to anaphylactic reactions from insect stings or certain foods. Even if you are not aware of a severe allergy within your family, having an EpiPen can save a life if someone experiences a severe reaction unexpectedly.

You'll want to include any specific medications required by you or your family in your kit as well.

Talk to your doctor about getting an extra prescription that can be placed in your first aid kit. The last thing you want to be doing is frantically searching for a necessary medication during an emergency situation.

Although it is illegal for a doctor to prescribe a controlled substance without an immediate need, antibiotics are not as strictly regulated. An extra stash of antibiotics could be a literal lifesaver if infection becomes serious.

Cephalexin (commonly marketed as Keflex) is an antibiotic that is especially good at treating staph infections that may be contracted after a serious laceration or puncture wound.

The last important component of any first aid kit is the case or bag that you keep it in.

If you were to follow this list completely you would need a rather large bag to carry everything. Whatever you choose to use, make sure it is durable and closes securely. You definitely don't want the contents of your first aid kit spilling all over the place during an emergency.

The ideal container will be waterproof or at least water resistant.

Many of the items contained within the kit are sensitive to water and can be rendered useless if exposed to wet conditions. You can buy specially built duffel bags designed for military use that have a waterproof liner built-in. These can be expensive but definitely not as expensive as your investment in

first aid equipment and gear.

Just like any other tool you rely on, your first aid kit requires periodic maintenance.

Maintenance of your kit includes taking a semiannual inventory and checking the expiration dates of any items that cannot be stored indefinitely.

Inventory is important in case someone grabs a piece of gear from the kit and forgets to replace it. By periodically checking the contents, you can be assured that the entire kit is available when called upon.

Some items, especially medications, can only be stored for a limited amount of time before they should be replaced. While checking your inventory, make notes of any expiration dates and write them on an index card that can be stored in the kit for quick reference.

If you know a certain medication will expire before your next inspection, take the initiative and replace it ahead of time. Antibiotics do not store very well, as an example, and their effectiveness is diminished greatly once the expiration period has been reached.

Have other family members help you do inventory so they can also become familiar with the contents of the kit and the potential uses for each item.

If you assemble the kit yourself, other family members may not be aware of the kit's content which greatly diminishes the usefulness of the first aid kit in an emergency.

Location, Location, Location

The location of your first aid kit is almost as important as the contents of it.

A first aid kit that is not easily accessible is practically useless. Your primary first aid kit should be located in a central area of your home and the location should be known to every family member.

If your budget allows, you should also consider creating multiple kits.

Not every first aid kit needs to be as large or complete as the primary kit, but each "satellite" kit should afford basic first aid items such as bandages and antiseptic solution.

Those readily available kits I mentioned at the beginning of this chapter could be an affordable option. These smaller kits can be placed in vehicles, in the garage, or anywhere else where people spend a lot of time and could get injured.

These portable first aid kits are also much easier to transport if an accident happens in a more remote location where the primary kit may not be available.

First Aid 101

When faced with an emergency situation, it's important to assess the situation properly before taking **any** action. Providing proper first aid to a victim is completely dependent on your ability to quickly and accurately assess the injury as well as any mitigating factors that could make the injury even more serious if not dealt with promptly.

Nine Simple Steps to Properly Assess Any Situation

Below, you will find nine simple steps that should be used anytime an emergency arises. Always refer to and follow these steps before proceeding with first aid treatment.

1. **Remain Calm**. It can be extremely difficult to avoid panicking when someone is injured. This is especially true when it is someone who know and/or care about. That said, you cannot be expected to make sound decisions when you aren't calm. Remaining calm also helps the victim by assuring them that everything will be OK. This psychological support is often enough to prevent the onset of shock when injuries are serious.

2. **The ABCs of Life Support**. The ABCs are the first things you need to check upon finding an injured person. This is especially true when you are unsure of the extent of injury or if you didn't see the event that caused the injury in the first place.

   a. Airways open. Ensure that the victim's airway is not obstructed and maintain this unobstructed airflow throughout treatment.

   b. Breathing restored. Check the victim for signs of breathing. Sometimes you cannot tell just by looking at the victim. In these instances, place your ear directly in front of the victim's mouth to listen and feel for breath. If the victim is not breathing, begin rescue breathing immediately (covered in Chapter Three).

   c. Circulation maintained. Check the victim's pulse. If no pulse (or an extremely faint pulse) is detected, begin cardiopulmonary resuscitation (CPR). Do not attempt CPR if not properly trained as this can lead to further injury. Fortunately, you will learn basic CPR in Chapter Three.

3. **Check for bleeding**. Scan the body for any signs of external bleeding. If bleeding is present, immediately apply direct pressure to the wound and elevate the area if possible.

4. **Look for signs of shock and fractured bones**. It isn't always readily apparent when a victim begins to go into shock, but common signs include feeling cold, profuse sweating, nonsensical speech, anxiety and lightheadedness. Shock makes treatment more difficult and should be addressed immediately by trying to keep the victim calm and comfortable. Also look for signs of broken bones at this time.

5. **Check for emergency medical identification**. If you are unsure of the health history of the victim, check the body for any identification that might indicate underlying medical conditions such as diabetes or

hemophilia (the inability of blood to clot normally). These medical cues can provide insight into how first aid treatment should continue and sometimes even explain the symptoms of a particular ailment.

6. **Call for professional assistance**. Although this isn't always possible in a survival situation, at least attempt to contact emergency medical personnel if the injury is beyond the scope of your training. You can also use smoke signals, three shots from a firearm or a safety whistle to signal others nearby that assistance is required.

7. **Loosen restrictive clothing**. Look for any clothing on the victim that could potentially restrict breathing or circulation and remove them immediately. This keeps the victim more comfortable and ensures maximum circulation of oxygenated blood throughout the body.

8. **NEVER give an unconscious victim anything by mouth**. The victim will likely choke if anything (water, food, medicine) is given orally. Wait until the victim has regained consciousness before administering any oral treatment.

9. **Do not move the victim**. Moving a victim, especially one with unknown injuries, could make the situation much worse. The only exception to this rule is if leaving the victim where they are could be life-threatening (such as lying on train tracks or in the middle of the road). In all other instances, leave the victim on location until the person is stabilized and the full extent of the injuries has been properly assessed.

In the next section, you will learn about some common first aid scenarios as well as ways to treat these conditions using supplies contained in your first aid kit.

Common First Aid Scenarios

Here are some examples of common situations that may require first aid and typical treatment options that help to mitigate further injury or complications:

Bleeding Wounds and Other Lacerations

Depending on the severity of the bleeding and its location, applying firm pressure to the immediate area will aid in the clotting process. If the bleeding is arterial, then a tourniquet may be required to prevent life-threatening blood loss.

Nosebleeds

A nosebleed is very rarely a life-threatening ailment. The exception is when the patient is a hemophiliac (a "bleeder"); a person unable to clot damaged blood vessels. Typically, pinching the nose shut is all that's required to stop a nosebleed.

Burns

Burns are typically categorized into first, second, or third degree classifications depending on the severity. First-degree burns typically do not require any special treatment while a third degree burn should be immediately wrapped to prevent the risk of serious infection. Burn creams do nothing for extremely severe burns and should be avoided.

Bites

Bee stings and spider bites are probably the most common biting injuries encountered during first aid treatment. These injuries are usually not serious but complications can arise because of allergic reactions. This condition is known as anaphylaxis and is deadly if left untreated. Snakebites can be more serious. The bite from a venomous snake can kill a human quickly. Wrapping the wound and keeping the patient relatively still will help to slow the spread of venom throughout the body.

Sudden collapse

A person may collapse for a number of reasons including respiratory distress, choking, or cardiac arrest among others. One of the staples of first aid treatment is commonly referred to as ABC – airway, breathing, and circulation. Assessing the ABCs of a patient can often shed light on the reasons for the collapse so that appropriate action can be taken.

Car accidents

Any accident involving a vehicle can often result in serious injuries including injuries to the spinal column. These victims should not be moved until appropriate equipment is available to stabilize the spinal column. Many basic first aid techniques can be administered while the victim is still in the vehicle.

Common injuries from car accidents include fractures, bleeding (both internal and external), neck/spinal injuries and an assortment of cuts, scrapes and abrasions.

Frostbite and Hypothermia

Frostbite occurs when human tissue begins to freeze due to exposure in extremely cold temperatures. Extremities such as the fingers, toes, ears and nose are most susceptible to frostbite. Minor frostbite can be treated easily by gently soaking the affected area(s) in warm water. Do not use direct heat (from a fire or stove) as this can lead to burns. In more extreme cases of frostbite, there is little that can be done from a first aid perspective and depending on the severity of the condition, the affected areas may ultimately require amputation.

The worst thing you can do when treating frostbite is to thaw a frozen area only to have it refreeze again. If you are unable to keep a frostbitten area warm, do not thaw the injury until such a time that it can be kept from refreezing.

Hypothermia occurs when the body's core temperature drops below 96°F. Symptoms of hypothermia include uncontrollable shivering, drowsiness, slurred speech and loss of coordination. These symptoms become increasingly obvious as the body continues to cool down.

Treating hypothermia is as simple as restoring the core body as quickly as possible. This can be done by placing the victim in a sleeping bag (or under a blanket) without clothing and having someone else (also naked) lay with the victim. The skin-to-skin contact helps warm the victim quickly. Assuming the victim is conscious, offering warm beverages also helps. It can take hours to raise the body temperature of someone suffering from hypothermia so be prepared to stay where you are for a long time while the victim recovers.

Severe Bleeding

When a victim is losing a lot of blood due to injury, quickly clean obvious dirt from the area and immediately apply direct pressure to the wound by placing sterile gauze over the area and pressing down as hard as possible. Depending on the extent of the injury, you may have to apply pressure for 30 minutes or more to control bleeding. If a major vein or artery has been opened, surgical scissors can be used to directly cut off blood supply to the affected area.

Do not put direct pressure onto the wound if an embedded object is present. Also, do not remove the embedded object as this usually causes even more bleeding. If a limb has been severely lacerated, you can also apply a tourniquet to the limb. Unfortunately, tourniquets often result in the amputation of an entire limb because the blood supply is almost entirely cut off during the process. Tourniquets should always be placed as close to the wound as possible for this reason and should only be considered when other options (namely direct pressure) haven't been effective.

You should also look for signs of internal bleeding which could signal an even more serious injury. Signs of internal bleeding include:

- Bleeding from any body opening including the ears, mouth, nose or anus.

- Vomiting or coughing up blood

- Unusual bruising

- Tender or swollen stomach

- Cold, clammy skin

- Shock in the absence of more obvious injuries

This is only a small sampling of the thousands of possible injuries you may encounter.

Fortunately, the techniques for administering proper first aid remain relatively unchanged throughout most of these situations. It's a good idea to enroll in various first aid classes to increase your knowledge and training in specialized techniques required for specific injuries.

Pain Relief

As someone trained in first aid techniques, there is another topic that needs to be covered: pain relief. Obviously, the first priority should always be stabilizing the victim, but keeping that person comfortable is also important component of first aid. How you manage pain for the victim depends on the nature of the injury, but there are some basic rules that help regulate pain in most common first aid scenarios.

Your first aid kit should include a supply OTC pain relievers such as acetaminophen (Tylenol) and nonsteroidal antiinflammatory agents (NSAIDS) including ibuprofen (Motrin). NSAIDS help to reduce swelling, but caution should be used when administering these medications to someone with a bleeding injury as NSAIDS tend to make blood thinner and less likely to clot. Once bleeding has stopped, however, Motrin is an excellent choice in most situations.

OTC pain relievers can also be used to keep a fever from getting dangerously high — making these medications a must-have for any first aid kit.

Instant cold packs are another way to reduce pain and swelling. Applying cold packs to bruises is especially effective at controlling swelling while providing some degree of pain relief to the victim.

If you have access to opiate pain killers (such as morphine), you can control pain in nearly any emergency. Unfortunately, most of these medications are considered controlled substances so obtaining access can be difficult. That said, you can sometimes find old military first aid kits that contain morphine via the Internet or a local military surplus store. Just realize that possessing these medications without a prescription is illegal in most cases so be careful if you choose to add them to your first aid repertoire.

There are also an assortment of topical ointments with pain relievers already mixed in. Examples include burn cream and bacitracin — both of which contain topical numbing agents that reduce pain when applied to a cut or burn.

If nothing else is available, alcohol can be used to reduce pain. Allowing a victim to consume a moderate amount of liquor will reduce their sensitivity to pain. Care must be exercised, however, because consuming too much alcohol can actually complicate medical conditions and make treatment more difficult. It's not a bad idea to keep a small bottle of alcohol (usually vodka or whiskey) in your first aid kit for times when other pain relief options are simply not effective.

Word of warning: if you do have access to opiate pain relievers, NEVER mix them with alcohol. The synergistic effects of these substances can create a dangerous situation for a victim as both substances work to depress the nervous system. In extreme cases, victims may lose the ability to breathe if their body becomes too depressed by the combination of opiates and alcohol.

Head & Neck Injuries

Head and neck injuries can be extremely difficult to diagnose without specialized equipment, but failure to address these injuries properly could lead to further injury including permanent paralysis or even death.

There are three types of head injuries:

- Injury to the scalp

- Injury to the brain

- Injury to the skull (commonly referred to as a skull fracture)

One of the first things you should look for when attempting to diagnose a head injury to is to look for signs of increased pressure within the skull. Symptoms of increased pressure include:

- Decreased mental function or strange responses to easy questions

- Erratic behavior or unexpected combativeness

- Unexplained nausea and/or vomiting

- Pupils that are not reactive to light (checked by shining a light into the eyes)

- Double vision

- Headaches

- Loss of memory

- Seizures

- Irregular breathing patterns

- Visible trauma to the head

You should always assume a spinal injury is present whenever a head injury is suspected. This means stabilizing both the head and neck (as described later in this section). Check for and monitor the ABCs like any other injury and be prepared for vomiting. If a victim begins to vomit, gently roll them into the recovery position while keeping the head and neck stabilized.

Also, be sure to treat the victim for shock by keeping them warm and comfortable. The only difference when a head injury is suspected is that you SHOULD NOT elevate the victim's legs as you normally would.

Stabilization of the Head and Neck

Whenever a spinal or head injury is suspected, it is imperative that the victim not be moved unless absolutely necessary to prevent further injury. At the bare minimum, use both hands to keep the neck and head stable during first aid treatment.

The use of a neck collar is even better as it allows you to maintain stability of the area while still having full use of your hands to perform first aid techniques.

If a victim needs to be moved for any reason, it should be done so in a way that prevents unnecessary movement to the affected area. The best way to do this is known as the log roll. Start by placing a stretcher (a makeshift stretcher works just as well as a purpose built one) next to the victim. Next, roll the entire body in one movement on the side and slide the stretcher into position underneath the victim. This requires at least two people to do safely.

Gently roll the victim back into position on the stretcher. When actually moving the person, be mindful of any movements that could place unnecessary stress on the head and neck.

Although it can be difficult to treat many head and neck injuries in the field, keeping the victim stabilized is the best way to prevent further injury while waiting for professional assistance to arrive.

Chapter Three: CPR & Rescue Breathing

Cardiopulmonary resuscitation (CPR) and rescue breathing are very important skills that every adult in your household should know how to do without a second thought. When a victim is unable to breathe or the heart has failed and blood is no longer circulating through the body as it should, death occurs within a matter of minutes. That's why it is essential to know these techniques — and know them well.

If you are fortunate enough to have an Automated External Defibrillator (mentioned in Chapter Two), you can often restart a failed heart without using CPR, but in every other instance, knowing how to artificially circulate oxygenated blood throughout the body is the difference between life and death in a survival situation.

Rescue breathing is done when the heart is still pumping blood — in other words, a strong pulse is detected. Rescue breathing is used when a victim is unable to pull oxygenated air into their bodies alone due to injury. By forcing air into his or her lungs, the heart is able to continue moving oxygenated blood throughout the circulatory system thereby greatly increasing the victim's chances of survival.

Rescue Breathing

If a victim is unconscious, one of the first things you want to do is check to see if the victim is breathing. As mentioned in Chapter Two, you can do this by placing your ear directly in front of the victim's mouth while both listening and feeling for exhaled air. If no breathing is detected, you must do two things before beginning rescue breathing. The first is to check the victim's airway for possible obstructions. Second, check the victim's pulse. If no pulse is present, skip rescue breathing and move right into CPR. If a pulse is detected, you may begin rescue breathing.

Start by making sure the victim is laying flat on his or her back. Gently tilt the head back enough to create a clear path from the mouth to the lungs. Ideally, your first aid contains a pocket mask or breathing barrier. This helps limit exposure to disease and provides a better seal. Place mask or barrier on the victim properly to create a seal.

If no mask is available, you can use use direct mouth-to-mouth contact so long as you can make a seal whereby air does not escape from between your lips and those of the victim during rescue breathing.

Now do two rescue breaths — each lasting approximately one second. You need to blow hard enough to force air into the victim's lungs, but not so hard as to possibly cause additional damage. Also, if the rescue breaths are too long, excess air will be forced into the victim's stomach which often results in vomiting. If the victim does begin to vomit, gently roll him or her onto their side (known as the recovery position) to allow the vomit out without obstructing the airway. Clean the mouth with your finger before resuming rescue breathing.

You should be watching the chest cavity while performing this technique. The chest should clearly rise when you breathe into the victim's lungs. If the chest does not clearly rise, tilt the head back slightly more and provide two more rescue breaths again watching to see if the chest cavity rises.

If the chest still doesn't rise, the victim is choking. The steps for handling unconscious choking are covered in the next section.

Assuming the chest cavity does rise, continue providing rescue breaths once every five seconds for adults (once every three seconds for children). Every two minutes, stop and confirm there is still a pulse before starting a new set of rescue breaths. You should stop rescue breathing when there is no pulse (CPR is needed), the victim begins breathing on their own or you become too exhausted to continue (in which case someone else can take over until professional help arrives or it is determined that the victim cannot recover).

Unconscious Choking Treatment

If during rescue breathing you realize the victim's chest cavity is not rising and falling in relation to the breaths you're providing, it means the victim has some sort of obstruction in the mouth, throat or trachea that is preventing air from entering the lungs.

After performing two more rescue breaths, perform five chest compressions. You should place your hands on top of one another right around the nipple line when performing this step. The compressions should be firm enough to forcefully dislodge any obstruction.

Now tilt the head back and hold the mouth open with your thumb. You should also hold the tongue with the same thumb to prevent the victim from choking on that and to aid in looking for the obstruction. Using a small flashlight, look carefully for anything that could be obstructing the airway. Run your finger through the mouth and throat feeling for an obstruction as well.

Continue this cycle until the obstruction has been located and removed.

Once the obstruction has been removed, begin providing rescue breaths as described in the previous section. Don't forget to check for a pulse every two minutes.

Cardiopulmonary Resuscitation (CPR)

CPR is required when a victim is no longer breathing or producing a detectable pulse. In other words, both the pulmonary system (lungs) and cardiovascular system (heart) are no longer working. The idea behind CPR is to simulate the actions of both the heart and lungs until the individual is able to once again perform these functions on their own. CPR provides oxygenated blood to vital organs including the brain while the person is unable to do it for themselves. When done properly, CPR has been proven to save lives that would otherwise be lost within a matter of minutes.

CPR is started the same way as rescue breathing. This action allows you to set up the mask or barrier before beginning CPR and more importantly, ensures that the airway if unobstructed before continuing. If the chest is not rising, follow the instructions for unconscious choking discussed in the previous section before continuing.

Check the victim for a pulse. Do this by placing two fingers in the groove of the victim's neck (do this for both children and adults). If no pulse is detected, start CPR immediately.

Start by administering two additional rescue breaths as described in previous sections.

Follow these rescue breaths with 30 chest compressions near the nipple line. This simulates the pumping of the heart and helps move oxygenated blood throughout the body. You should strive to create a rhythm that is approximately 100 compressions per minute (although you are only doing 30). This is a relatively fast pace but is required to move blood in an efficient manner. You should aim to compress the sternum about 1/3 the width of the chest cavity.

Keep in mind that sometimes the amount of pressure required to do chest compressions correctly can break rib bones. Although this is not ideal, a broken rib is much easier to treat after the person has recovered than the victim not recovering at all.

Perform two more rescue breaths followed by 30 more chest compressions. Continue this cycle until the victim has a pulse and begins breathing or until you are too exhausted to perform CPR anymore (at which time another trained adult should take over).

It's worth noting that an AED is a much better way to resuscitate someone if available. CPR can be used while an AED is located (most public places have at least one available). Once the AED is available, immediately stop CPR and use the AED instead.

Another thing to keep in mind is that many modern CPR classes are no longer teaching rescue breaths in conjunction with chest compressions when performing CPR. Although doing both has worked in many instances, some experts believe that rescue breaths can do more harm than good and advise that CPR consist only of chest compressions until an AED can be found, emergency medical personnel arrive or it becomes apparent that the victim will not recover.

Conventional CPR (with rescue breaths) can be performed by two people to make it less exhausting. One person does the chest compressions while the other performs rescue breathing immediately after. Then both people change positions allowing both individuals to recover from doing chest compressions (which, when done correctly, is extremely tiring because of the amount of force required).

Once the victim does recover, gently rotate them into the recovery position (on their side).

Using one (or more) of these techniques is often the difference between life and death when serious injuries occur. The best way to master these techniques is to enroll in a local CPR class held by the Red Cross or another organization. These classes provide life-size dummies complete with a "working" chest cavity that rises when performing rescue breaths. This is a very effective way to master the skills required to perform these life-saving techniques under the guidance of a trained professional.

Chapter Four: Survival Medicine

As we discussed in Chapter One, there is a definite difference between first aid and survival medicine. While many of the same concepts apply to both, our definition of survival medicine means that we need to cultivate solutions that can be used for long periods of time or in situations where your entire first aid kit isn't available.

Remember how we talked about using a tree branch as a splint? That's what this chapter is about. But it's also about a lot more than that. It's about using improvisation and sustainable techniques to create treatment and medicine options that won't necessarily be available in a long-term survival situation.

If you get anything from this chapter, it should be that in order to provide alternative medicine to your family you need to change your perspective about healthcare and medicine in general.

We live in a society that has been conditioned to go to the doctor for everything from minor scrapes to common colds.

Cutting-edge medical science is something we view as a distant corporate entity full of mystery that provides all sorts of medication to our local pharmacies; sometimes at astronomical costs.

We are a society that has lost the homeopathic remedies used by our ancestors for thousands of years. In fact, society has become so jaded that in many circles herbal medicine is viewed as barbaric or unsophisticated… something that is best left for people to practice on their own but certainly not something worthy of mainstream acceptance.

Pharmaceutical companies have become the "cure-all" for everything that ails us.

If you have a stomach ache – you purchase Pepto-Bismol. If you have a cough, you buy cough medicine. If you have a cold, you might purchase cold medicine to help with the many symptoms associated with feeling under the weather.

But it doesn't stop there.

If you have a cut, you look for ointments such as bacitracin to ward off infection and quicken healing times.

For skin care, we often resort to lotions and creams with many chemical names that are simply too difficult to pronounce. Even mental health is addressed with pills in our modern society.

To become truly resilient, we must take action. We need to take control of our own health care to ensure longevity.

It is a two-part process requiring proactive preventive care as well as treatment when injury or illness strikes.

We have to realize that not every minor ailment requires professional medical attention. I'm not here to devalue the extraordinary knowledge and training of medical staff. Rather, I am simply pointing out what may appear obvious to some – many people have become so dependent on the health care system that even minor injuries cannot be addressed at home.

Fortunately, this is simple to change. Much of it comes simply from changing your perspective regarding healthcare and medicine in general.

We should look to adopt a mindset where professional medicine becomes a last resort after we have exhausted all efforts to treat common illnesses at home.

Please don't take out your health insurance card and cut it into shreds just yet. Doctors provide an invaluable service to the community.

The point is simply to illustrate that we can approach sustainable healthcare solutions designed to meet long-term survival needs. After all, our future is unknown and the effects of societal collapse could leave modern medicine as a thing of the past.

In this chapter, we will look at some common alternative medicine techniques that can be practiced at home. By growing your own herbs, you may be surprised by how well-equipped you are to provide medical treatments for a variety of ailments.

Not only does this save you money on commercial medicine, it also makes you more resilient; more able to survive in any circumstance.

The Benefits of Alternative Medicine

When we think of alternative medicine, what comes to mind?

Often, it is herbs and other plants being administered in place of chemical compounds developed in a lab.

The problem is that society has been led to believe that these chemical cures surpass the abilities of natural treatment options. In some cases they do. Technology has afforded society new solutions that were simply not available in centuries past.

With the billions of dollars that are spent in the pharmaceutical industry each year, it's no wonder why pharmaceutical companies would have you believe that their cures are more effective.

What they don't tell you is that in the United States as much as 70% of all new medicinal drugs have been developed from natural sources.

What this means as we strive to become more independent is that we can harness much of this same technology in our own backyards.

Many home herbal remedies can be created from simple, easy to grow plants. These plants are right at home in a backyard garden or even in a windowsill herb garden if that's the only space you have available.

Regardless of where you choose to grow your herbs, there are thousands of varieties offering different cures and preparation methods.

The only thing we need is a little additional knowledge about common preparation methods and herbs that can be effectively used to treat a variety of ailments.

With that knowledge, we are able to create treatment options of our own.

Herbal remedies are often much less expensive than commercial counterparts. Even a windowsill herb garden can provide enough medicine to save you hundreds of dollars a year in OTC drug purchases.

Everything from the common cold to digestive problems can usually be addressed effectively using plants that are easy to grow practically anywhere.

Another benefit of herbal remedies is the sustainability inherent to relying on them. It's no secret that the dollar loses value all the time and necessary items become more expensive almost daily. The day could come where even a bottle of Tylenol may be out of financial reach for most of society.

In fact, stores could cease to exist altogether – leading to zero availability of OTC medications at all.

Herbal remedies can be grown, prepared, and administered right from home. There is no need for a doctor or a hospital to address many common injuries and illnesses.

The sustainability of herbal remedies has been proven for centuries. Even in North America, natives have relied on herbal remedies to cure a variety of illnesses successfully. They did this without pharmaceutical laboratories or expensive equipment.

We can do this too. In fact, we need to do this if we want to lessen our reliance on commercial medicine; an industry that could fail at any time.

Delivery Methods

The delivery method refers to the way a specific treatment is administered. There are a variety of ways to administer herbal remedies depending on specific ailments and the properties of the plant matter being used.

Let's take a look at some of the most common delivery methods and how they are created at home.

Infusions

Infusions are one of the easiest delivery methods to create at home. An infusion is nothing more than a cup of tea.

Infusions provide a quick and easy way to consume the beneficial ingredients of many plants without the need for lengthy processes or other ingredients.

To make infusion, you will need approximately 30 g of fresh leaves or flowers or approximately 15 g of dried material.

A teapot is the easiest way to make infusion although a glass bowl can be used instead. If you are using a bowl, make sure that you cover it so the essential oils do not evaporate from your infusion. Let the tea steep for between 8 – 10 minutes before straining the solids from the liquid and consuming.

Infusions are also commonly used when making creams and lotions.

Some people also create infusions that are designed to be poured into the bathtub for an herbal soak. If the flavor of the tea is not to your liking, you can add honey or sugar to make it slightly more palatable.

Infusions do not store well and should be consumed the same day they are made. You can make a batch in the morning and keep it refrigerated throughout the day but anything left over in the evening should be discarded and a fresh infusion created.

Decoctions

A decoction is similar to an infusion except the process takes longer because the plant matter tends to be tougher.

Examples might include roots, twigs, seeds, or bark. All of these materials will require longer soak times to successfully extract the ingredients.

To make a decoction, wash and cut up the roots, bark, or other materials. This exposes a larger surface area and makes extraction more effective.

In a pan, put your plant matter and add 500 mL of water for every 30 g of fresh plant material or 15 g of dried material. Cover the pan, bring it to a boil, and then allow it to simmer for approximately 30 minutes.

Slightly longer cooking times may be required for extremely tough roots or bark. Strain the organic material left over from the cooking process before consuming the decoction. Decoctions are also used in the making of lotions and creams.

Storing decoctions is very similar to storing infusions. They are designed to be consumed the same day they are made but can be stored in a refrigerator for approximately a 24-hour period before they should be discarded.

Infused Oils

Infused oils are used as massage and bath oils but more importantly – they are the base from which you can make creams, rubs, and salves. Infused oils capture the flavor, colors, and essential compounds of the plants.

Some herbal oils are also used in cooking or as a salad dressing.

To make infused oil, fill a glass jar with a screw-on top approximately ¾ full of plant material that has been crushed lightly.

Pour over your oil of choice but make sure that the plant material is completely covered in oil. If plant material is not submerged in oil, it can grow mold during the extraction process.

Seal the jar and leave it in a warm spot for approximately 2 weeks. Shake the bottle every 1 – 2 days and be sure to push down any plant material that is no longer submerged in the oil.

After the two week time period has elapsed, strain the liquid into a bottle.

When making infused oils, the base oil you use is dependent on the intended use of the infused oil.

If the oil is going to be used for a cream or lotion, choose a light, non-greasy vegetable oil. Sunflower oil and grapeseed oil work well for this.

If the oil is going to be consumed, use the same oils that you normally would when cooking.

Since infused oils typically take approximately two weeks for a successful extraction, consider using this quick solution if you need the oil immediately.

Place the plant matter into a glass bowl and cover with oil before placing the bowl above a pot of boiling water.

Cook the mixture, covered, for approximately one hour or until the oil has taken on the color of the herb. Strain the liquid and bottle in the same way you would after the two-week extraction period.

Although this method may not produce the same richness and complete extraction, it is a quick solution if an infused oil is needed right away.

Infused oils will typically last for between 6 – 12 months if they are stored in a cool, dark place in tightly sealed container.

Vinegars

Vinegars can be made from plant matter exactly the same way that infused oils are. Typically, herbal vinegars might be made into a daily tonic but also work well in compresses, as mouthwashes, and as a hair product.

As with infused oils, make sure the plant matter is fully submerged in the vinegar to avoid mold or rot.

Cider or white wine vinegar can be used effectively. Storage times are also similar and herbal vinegars will usually have a shelf life between six months and one year.

Tinctures

A tincture is when you use alcohol to extract the active ingredients of a plant. The potency of alcohol makes it much more effective than oil or vinegar as an extraction agent.

It is especially useful on tougher plant materials like roots and resins. Tinctures have a much longer shelf life as the alcohol acts as a preservative. Tinctures also tend to be much more concentrated than infused oils, vinegars, or other solutions.

To make a tincture, fill a glass jar approximately ¾ full with plant matter and cover with your choice of alcohol.

Although you can use any alcohol rated at 80 proof (40% alcohol) or above, vodka is usually best because it is colorless and nearly tasteless.

Making sure that all of the plant material is submerged, seal the jar and store in a dark place at room temperature for about one month.

If you choose to make a tincture out of "softer" materials (such as leaves and flowers) the extraction process will not take nearly this long. The one month time frame is more appropriate for roots, resins, and other tough plant matter.

Shake the glass jar once every couple of days during the extraction process. Strain the liquid into small, dark glass bottles for storage.

Tinctures can last for two years or more if stored in cool, dark places. The colored glass prevents the alcohol from evaporating and the tincture will last much longer as a result.

You may not want to use alcohol in your tinctures due to personal choice or if you are creating a tincture for a child.

Glycerites

A glycerite is essentially a tincture that uses glycerin instead of alcohol. Glycerin has a sweet and syrupy taste making it perfect for use in children's remedies. Please note that glycerin is not as effective as an extraction agent – this means that the final product will be slightly less concentrated and have a shorter shelf life.

To make a glycerite, fill a glass jar ¾ full of plant material and fully submerge in glycerin. This method will not work well on extremely tough plant material do to glycerin's inability to break down the ingredients.

Leaves and flowers will be the most effective way to make glycerites and these should be allowed to soak for approximately 2 weeks.

Glycerites do not require dark-colored bottles like tinctures but expect them to have a shelf life of only about one year.

Gels

Gels are used as jellies and in skin preparations because they have good astringent properties. An example might be aloe vera gel used to treat sunburn. They are also used to make hair and aftershave gels.

Gels are made by adding gelatin or another clear thickener to the recipe and stirring until the mixture thickens to a gel consistency. Powdered vegetable gelatin dissolves easily and can be purchased from the baking section of most supermarkets.

A simple gel can be created by pouring approximately 100 mL of a plant infusion into a pan with a small amount (about 6 g) of gelatin.

Follow the directions on the gelatin you choose for the exact amount you should be using. Stir the mixture until the powdered gelatin dissolves and then heat for a couple of minutes while continuously stirring until a gel is formed.

You can also add infused oils for additional medicinal properties.

Gels do not store well at all. They can be kept in the refrigerator but should be used within approximately 2 days if they are being consumed.

Gels for topical use can be kept in the refrigerator for about four weeks.

Ointments, Salves and Balms

Ointments, salves, and balms are oil and wax preparations made to various consistencies depending on the application.

An ointment is usually thinner than a salve and typically applied over large areas of the body. If you have ever used Vick's Vapor Rub for a cough, this is a perfect example of an ointment.

Salves and balms are typically thicker and waxier and are usually designed for use on specific areas such as cut or rash.

To make a basic ointment, put 300 mL of infused oil into a glass bowl with 25 g of beeswax. If you purchase solid wax, break it into small pieces. You can even use beeswax candles (as long as they are 100% beeswax).

Gently heat the mixture by placing the bowl over a pan of simmering water and stir gently until all the wax is melted.

Pour the melted wax into a jar before it begins to solidify. If you need to make a thicker mixture, add more beeswax. Conversely, a thinner mixture can be created by adding more infused oil.

All of these mixtures have a good shelf life and will last for a year or more without any special storage considerations.

Creams

A slightly more complicated process can be used to create creams.

Creams are useful because they provide moisture to skin and allow plant ingredients to be quickly absorbed. Creams are basically a combination of oil and water which is held together with an emulsifier. A combination of beeswax and emulsifying wax seems to work best.

To make a cream, put 40 mL of infused oil into a glass bowl with 6 teaspoons of emulsifying wax and 2

teaspoons of beeswax.

Like ointments, heat the bowl over a pan of simmering water until the wax is completely dissolved. Now pour 250 mL of warm water into the bowl slowly while stirring vigorously.

Once the mixture begins to melt, remove it from heat and continue stirring while the cream cools. Failure to continue stirring at this point could result in the oil and water separating.

The cream can now be spooned into a resealable jar for storage. Creams do take some practice to get right. Failure to mix the ingredients properly often results in a cream that fails to emulsify well. Practice makes perfect on this one.

Creams can last for approximately 2 months in the refrigerator although they may need to be stirred from time to time as the oil and water begin to separate during storage.

Common Ailments and Cures

Attempting to cover every possible ailment and associated herbal remedy in this guide would be futile.

There are thousands of herbal remedies available and a number of ways to prepare them depending on the specific application.

Furthermore, the sheer number of ailments that can be cured using herbal medicine makes discussing every situation impossible.

Instead, we will focus on a few groups of common ailments and some herbs that can be used to cure them.

Digestive Problems

- Angelica

- Caraway seeds

- Ginger

- Fennel

- Marshmallow

- Peppermint

- Slippery elm

All of these herbs can be used to create remedies for stomach aches, cramping, and general digestive health. These remedies need to be consumed so infusions, decoctions, and glycerites are usually the most effective. Tinctures may not be appropriate because alcohol can aggravate many digestive related problems.

Respiratory Problems

- Echinacea

- Elderberries

- Eucalyptus

- Ginger

- Goji berries

- Nettles

- Onions

- Garlic

Especially for colds and the flu, Echinacea and Eucalyptus are excellent for boosting immune system health. Infusions are very effective. Ointments that can be placed under the nose for inhalation also work well. Especially for children, a vaporizer with infused oils is an effective treatment option.

Dermatological Problems

- Aloe Vera

- Chamomile

- Chickweed

- Pot marigold

- Plantain

- St. John's wort

- Tea tree

- Witch hazel

Skin problems such as cuts, rashes, bruises, burns, insect bites, and even eczema can be addressed by herbal creams, ointments, and balms. A gel made from aloe vera is excellent for treating the symptoms of sunburn and dry skin.

Kid-specific Treatments

Children benefit from all the same herbal remedies as adults but can often be much pickier about the types of things they are willing to consume. You should have a supply of sweet or fruity tasting plants to make treatment more enjoyable such as:

- Bilberries

- BlackBerries

- Blackcurrants

- Chamomile

- Elderberries

- Honeysuckle

- Mint

- Rose hip

- Ginger

These flavorful plants can be added to other remedies to mask the taste of unpalatable mixtures. Some of these plants, such as ginger, are great remedies alone. Ginger can be used effectively against travel sickness.

Muscular & Joint Problems

- Chili

- Eucalyptus

- Ginger

- Horseradish

- Licorice

- Turmeric

Topical treatments such as ointments and balms made from these herbs can relieve sore muscles and the symptoms of stiff joints.

Emotional Problems

- Gotu kola

- Lemon balm

- St. John's wort

- Vervain

- Ginseng

- Rose root

There are a large number of herbs that have been proven to promote mental health by increasing the amount of naturally occurring neurotransmitters (like serotonin) in the body. Infusions are typically the easiest way to consume these plants.

This is only a small sampling of the many illnesses and ailments that can be cured using herbs grown in your home.

Natural supplement stores are an excellent place to learn more about cures for particular illnesses. Spend a few hours walking through a store and just read the bottles. Often, these bottles explain exactly what each herb is used for and the remedies can often be replicated at home.

Figuring out what herbal remedies work and which ones don't is often a trial and error process. Fortunately, there usually aren't any negative side effects associated with trying different things until you find something that works.

This may sound rudimentary, but think about your last visit with the doctor.

Often, they will try a particular medication and instruct you to contact them if your symptoms don't improve. Since there are so many cures available for most ailments, there are bound to be some that work better than others and herbal medicine is no exception.

Top 10 Herbs You Should Be Growing Right Now

This topic is sure to invoke debate.

Anytime you have a "Top 10" list, there will always be people saying "well, what about…" or "why didn't you include…?" The herbs in this list have been chosen for their various medical properties and because they are considered easy to grow in just about any backyard environment.

Certainly, there are other herbs that may be best suited for your individual needs but the following list represents diversity and simplicity:

Calendula – Also known as pot marigold, calendula has antifungal, antiseptic, and wound healing properties. The petals of these orange flowers are excellent for natural cosmetic products and diaper creams.

Cilantro – Cilantro is commonly used as a garnish, but it is also a powerful digestive aid and can help the body cleanse itself of heavy metals and other toxic agents.

Lemon Balm – The oils and tannins in lemon balm have a relaxing effect on the stomach and the nervous system. When turned into a topical agent, the herb can also fight off viruses such as herpes simplex.

Peppermint – In addition to being popular as a flavor additive in candies, gum, and toothpaste, peppermint is excellent at relieving digestive discomfort including indigestion and vomiting when consumed as an infusion (tea). When used topically, it is also effective at soothing sore muscles

and joints.

Rosemary – Rosemary is an excellent alternative to caffeine. It works as a stimulant by bringing more oxygen to your brain and is much healthier to consume than copious amounts of coffee. Energy, optimism, memory, and concentration can all be improved by regularly consuming rosemary.

Mullein – This plant contains expectorant properties that can help to heal bronchial respiratory infections. Consuming an infusion made from the leaves of this plant works as an excellent cough medicine.

Thyme – Thyme has been used for centuries for a variety of ailments. The plant has many antibacterial and antiseptic properties that can help to prevent colds. The tannins in the plant may also help to relieve mild diarrhea symptoms.

Lavender – In addition to its pleasant fragrance, lavender is known to alleviate stress and work as a mild antidepressant. It can also be used in cream form to treat sunburn and acne.

German Chamomile – Chamomile can be used to treat colic, emotional stress, infections, and stomach disorders. It is especially useful for children's remedies and is best consumed as an infusion.

Garlic – Garlic has been proven to reduce the risk of contracting certain types of cancer, it has cardiovascular benefits, and it has antiseptic qualities as well. It also tastes great in a number of foods.

There are hundreds of other herbs you should consider growing in addition to those listed. The amount of space you have and your experience in growing herbs will play a role in just how many plants you decide to grow.

Growing Herbs at Home

One of the best parts about growing herbs at home is that many of them grow naturally as weeds.

This makes them extremely robust and easily grown in a variety of locations depending on the amount of space you have available and other plants you may be growing in the vicinity.

For the purposes of this report, let's assume that you have a limited amount of backyard space which is currently being used to produce fruits and vegetables.

That leaves little room to grow herbs. The good news is that most of the herbs we have talked about so far can be easily grown in a small windowsill herb garden.

Alternatively, a vertical garden is an excellent way to grow a large number of herbs in a very small space.

Just like any other plant you grow, each herb will have specific sunlight, watering, and soil requirements that you should take the time to research before starting.

All the herbs we have discussed in this guide are extremely easy to grow in a variety of conditions, eliminating the need for expensive setups or lots of preparatory work.

A vertical garden can be set up for less than $40 and represents the perfect opportunity for growing a medicinal herb garden.

Not only does a vertical garden take up much less space, but you tend to have more control over the nutrients that each plant receives. This means faster and larger yields.

A vertical herb garden made out of 4" PVC pipe can easily accommodate all 10 herbs listed in our Top 10 list.

Remember that most herbs can be harvested and dried for use in remedies in the future without any adverse effects on the potency of the product. There are some exceptions to this, such as lemon balm, which tends to lose potency after about six months of storage.

The point is that an herb garden does not have to take up a lot of space or hours of your time to be effective.

Small herb gardens are typically all that's required to begin creating herbal remedies that ultimately save you money and unnecessary trips to the doctor's office or the drugstore and these techniques work just as well now as they will in a future long-term survival situation.

Conclusion

Every effort has been made to make this guide easy to use in a variety of emergency situations; however, the importance of proper hands-on training cannot be stressed enough. Most first aid classes are free of charge and can be completed in a few hours over the weekend.

I urge each and every one of you to look into the availability of these classes in your area. Not only will you learn how to apply the techniques discussed in this guide, you will learn them under the supervision of a certified instructor.

Remember that the basic principle of any first aid response should be maintaining the ABCs for the victim while treating any wounds simultaneously. Failure to keep blood and oxygen flowing through the victim's body almost always leads to certain death.

The combination of first aid and alternative medicinal techniques that work well in long-term survival situations are essential to any survival plan. Whether you are stranded on a weekend camping trip or hiding in the wilderness following societal collapse, these techniques work — but only when you take the time to understand and practice them.